The Future of Chiropractic Business
Michael Goetsch D.C

A Note from the Author

The Future of Chiropractic Business was written to benefit the entire chiropractic profession. We are at a unique point in our profession's life cycle, and we are going to have to make some difficult decisions about the future course of our profession. I am uniquely concerned about how our profession is run from a business standpoint which is why I began my journey in studying and researching the business of chiropractic and how to better it.

At the beginning of this process, I only sought to find ways to better my own practice and increase my patient base, yet as I delved further into the flaws in how the chiropractic business operated where I worked; I realized that these flaws were universal in chiropractic. I was new to the profession, and these issues were glaring to me, and I wondered why no one had tried to identify or fix these problems. I soon realized that many chiropractors that I talked with were nervous about "rocking the boat" too much in chiropractic. They were comfortable with where the profession currently was, and didn't want to change.

After two years of research, this book became necessary to write so that we, together as chiropractors, can address these issues in our profession. This book is meant to invoke a conversation and inspire the action necessary to change our profession so that it can be the healthcare leader in the 21st century.

Contents

1

Introduction

The chiropractic profession is on the verge of total collapse, regardless of how successful your private practice may be today. Many chiropractors are feeling very comfortable right now because their practice is seeing record numbers and profits. Private practices have exploded all over the country, and most chiropractors have been able to strike a nerve in their communities which has given financial stability and success for many today. Unfortunately, we are enjoying a false sense of security within the profession, and it will not be long before we feel the effects across the entire profession.

The potential threat to our profession is not going to come from the medical profession trying to disparage our profession, or even from a lack of patients who seek our care. This problem is an internal struggle that has manifested itself many ways throughout our profession. That problem our entire profession has is the resistance to change, even when all indicators tell us to do so. I am not talking about the way in which we treat, because the chiropractic adjustment, regardless of technique, is the single-most effective procedure in healthcare today. I am referring to our profession's resistance to change or modify the way in which we do business in chiropractic.

Why is the only way you can be successful in our profession is to open a private practice in hopes of growing it into a reputable and profitable business? Why is that the only way new graduates can come into the profession and actually make any money to pay off student loans? Because no one has innovated any new ways to do business within chiropractic. We see private practice after private practice getting started all across America and none of them are truly any different at the fundamental level in how they are doing business or why they are in business.

Chiropractic will never grow if we refuse to take a long hard look at how we do business today, and once we see our faults, properly modify our business strategies. I have reached out to the leaders in our profession, from presidents of chiropractic universities to well-known and successful chiropractors, to give me their solution to our lack of growth within the profession and none of them have even considered that there is a problem to address. After feeling discouraged that our leaders had no motivation to understand the challenges we face in chiropractic today, I took this responsibility upon myself to identify and offer my solution to the business problems we face in chiropractic today. This book lays out my journey from identifying the problem to offering the best solution.

Chiropractic Facts and Figures

Chiropractors have seen tremendous success within America, which substantiates the profession's growth at tremendous rates with the number of new applicants pursuing a Doctor of Chiropractic (D.C.) degree every year. There is a current influx of 2,500 new chiropractors every year adding to the current slate of 77,000 chiropractors who already practice within the United States. The Bureau of Labor Statistics is projecting a 17% increase of new chiropractors by 2024. If these projections hold true, there will be approximately 90,000 chiropractors practicing in 2024. Some chiropractors will retire in this time, but growth is far greater than those dropping out of the profession. With all factors being addressed, there will approximately be 85,000 chiropractors with licenses in the United States. With all this projected growth, many analysts see chiropractic as a great career opportunity, but they fail to see the fundamental problem within chiropractic that has caused the profession to stall in terms of growth fiscally.

Per the Bureau of Labor Statistics, the average chiropractic salary is $66,720 which includes everyone from clinicians, associates, teachers, and other career paths that a Doctor of Chiropractic could hold. With the current 77,000 chiropractors, salaries equal to $5.13 billion dollars (37%) of the total income of the entire industry. Although this is a great percentage for doctors of chiropractic to be taking home, there are a few causes for concern if the numbers that are shown in the previous paragraph are examined. With the profession's projected growth of 17% by the year 2024, the gross income of the entire industry would need to increase by almost $3 billion dollars to remain at the same percentage of money in chiropractic salaries. A three billion-dollar growth in this same time frame would be a 21.4% increase on the current gross total of the entire profession. Which is not impossible, but usually the doctors who have the practices capable of growing large patient bases are the ones who have been in practice the longest, and are about ready to retire. The new doctors that are coming into the profession require time to mature relationships and build trust in their communities before they can begin to grow a respectable patient base. This problem shows that no matter how successful chiropractic is currently, it is heading for a big collapse when there is a large influx of new doctors, yet not a large influx of new patients. This will be a unique challenge that the profession will face in the next 5-7 years; to grow by $3 billion dollars to stay at current trends or become so over-utilized in every city that competition will completely dry up any profits there currently are enjoyed in chiropractic. Excessive competition in an industry creates a crisis for profits, as seen in the restaurant business. With a plethora of many different restaurants, investors hesitate to fund a "new restaurant" because of the challenge to differentiate itself in that industry. The same is true of chiropractic today. There is no way a chiropractor can pay off his student loan debt, keep his family financially stable, and continue to keep his practice open for business to make a profit in the market conditions within chiropractic.

A crisis within the profession is already brewing, and no one has tried to identify the problem or the solution. The entire profession must understand that if we do absolutely nothing, there will be ruin to the healing profession of chiropractic. We cannot sustain our growth within the profession, especially while the medical profession seeks to sweep up our patient base and the insurance companies look to lower our reimbursement rates. There are too many angles of attack upon chiropractic. We must realize that if we do nothing we will be pushed back into the recesses of history, which is an option, or we can come together to blaze a new path in which future chiropractors can follow for years to come.

2

Introductory Concepts for Chiropractors

What is our WHY?

"People don't buy what you do; they buy why you do it."-Simon Sinek

When Simon Sinek coined those famous words in his book *Start with Why*, he did not realize the vast implications it would mean for businesses all over the world. Many chiropractic businesses began with the motivation of treating as many patients as possible, hopefully seeing improvement, and making some good money in the process. Though those three motivations are not wrong, they do not inspire anyone to "buy in" to what chiropractors do. We've run ourselves ragged in this profession with ways to increase all three of those goals, and to what success? The profession, as a whole, is struggling to do each of those three things, and the problem is not in what we are doing, it's in the WHY we are doing it.

If your only motivation is to make more money than you can stop reading this book because that is not what this new business model seeks to do, although it is a result of the changes that we will make. If we only sought to change within the profession to make money, we can forget that this book was ever written. These changes are certainly beneficial, but they will only become necessary if we understand our reasoning (WHY) for altering the business model of the profession.

If our WHY within the profession isn't to make money, then what possibly could it be? I want to lay out a one sentence summary of what we must endeavor to do as a profession to properly execute the future success of our profession. Our why must be, **"To inspire our patients (through how we treat and what we promote as chiropractors) to pursue a healthier life for themselves."** Our focus cannot be on ourselves as the doctors. To effectively reach the world with a healthier alternative, the focus must solely be placed on the patients. Once we have created an environment where the patient is in control of his/her health, then chiropractic will be in the best place to serve those people. In medicine, we try to force our way of thinking down the patient's throat and almost guilt them into coming to see us. We, as chiropractors, do screenings to show the patient that they have some issues going on with their spine and that the chiropractor is the only one who could properly fix those issues. Medical doctors are guilty of this as well, they convey that they are the final answer on all things regarding health and that whatever an M.D says supersedes any other medical professional's opinion. This leaves patients feeling cornered and obligated to seek care from a doctor, when they should feel inspired and motivated to seek care for themselves. When patients are motivated to take control of their health, then we have truly done our job as chiropractors.

Another quote that inspired me as I was thinking about my true motivation for displaying this idea was from Guy Kawasaki. He articulated, "The companies that are successful, they start out to make meaning, not to make money." Guy spoke from his experiences of working with Steve Jobs. To Jobs, making the Macintosh computer or the entire Apple brand was not about making money; it was about changing the world through personal computers. Jobs and Wozniak were unaware of their future financial success by making their first Apple computer, but they did have a vision for how much progress they would create. Because of "making meaning", they created one of the most profitable and influential companies in the world.

Within this book, I will use terms that only reflect the business aspect of chiropractic, but our goal is to increase patient care by streamlining the model by which we administer our care. This entire business plan may do absolutely nothing in increasing profits within the chiropractic profession, but it will increase patient care quality. **With groups of our brightest minds working together in centers all over the world, chiropractic will take the lead as the foremost experts on HEALTHcare.** These centers will focus on HEALTHcare, because we must create an environment in our centers where the patients feel inspired and motivated to live a healthy life for themselves without reliance on doctors or pharmaceuticals.

I mentioned in that last sentence that we cannot create an environment where the patients RELY on us as the chiropractor to make them better or healthy again. That may sound like a horrible business strategy, but it is how we must make a difference in this world. Educated patients are far more fulfilling than needy patients who can't remain healthy without our help as doctors. We must stop thinking that the patients are helpless without us and focus our culture on educating those patients on how to remain healthy. I am convinced that if we focus 100% on empowering the patient, that the business side of things will take care of itself. **Our focus must be on changing the healthcare industry.**

We can create that culture at our centers across the world, but it starts with coming together as a profession toward that common goal. The following chapters will highlight just how unity within our profession will create a future where we can effectively change lives.

We have established our WHY as a profession, which was step one to accomplishing our goal. For the rest of this book, I will show HOW we change, through a unified chiropractic business model, that will change the entire industry.

Where are we as a profession right now? According to the latest Palmer College of Chiropractic Gallup Poll, chiropractors see approximately 12% of the population of the United States on a consistent basis, with 25% saying they have gone to a chiropractor before. These numbers are great for a business if it were retaining 12% of the population; but for a healthcare industry, these numbers are abysmal at best. Every year chiropractors are dropping out of the profession to find other jobs that can pay their bills. Chiropractic students are forced into associateships and contracts that seldom allow them to experience financial freedom after school. Doesn't this seem backwards for a healthcare profession? After all, we have one of the most powerful secrets to help people with their health and avoid serious health issues throughout their life. With this amazing potential, why are we floundering as a profession with our scope of practice being threatened each year, and with our bottom lines growing thinner and thinner each month. How did we get here?

Chiropractors got into this position because we never sought to grow together as a profession. Instead, individual chiropractors went out on their own and began to grow their private practice with the mindset of helping the largest number of people. This was the perfect model in the late 1900's-practices were booming, reimbursement rates were high and patients were getting well. Then the profession plateaued and has been at a standstill ever since. Our growth as a profession has stopped, while the number of chiropractors entering the profession has grown every year at alarming rates. Per the Bureau of Labor Statistics, we are projected to grow by 17% by the year 2024. That's about 8,000 more chiropractors that we will be forced to accommodate in this profession in the next few years. If we stay at the current 12% of patient base that we have, there will be more chiropractic practices failing, higher defaults on student loans, and more physicians dropping out of the profession altogether. There has to be something that can be done to grow our profession past that 12% and create a new era for the chiropractic profession. Good news, there is a way. Throughout this book, I am going to prove with simple numbers and examples how we as a profession can band together and create a market-share that is thriving for years to come.

Law of Diffusion of Innovation

The law of diffusion of innovation is a helpful model to show how any product, service, or good can view how it is breaking into the market. It is a curve that gives a breakdown of potential buyers, and this can be easily applied to the chiropractic market.

The first 2.5% are the *innovators*. These are the ground-breaking pioneers, doctors of our profession today-the ones that are discovering new techniques and skills under the umbrella of our chiropractic profession. These are the gentlemen and ladies that have started and practice techniques like the Cox technique, Functional neurology, Clinical Neuroscience, Torque Release Technique, Motion Palpation Institute, Gonstead, Diversified and so many others. These are the select men and women who through hard work find ways to treat the human body that so many medical professionals seem to overlook or think impossible. These people understand chiropractic and are patients of chiropractors, since they blaze the trail that the rest of us follow.

The next 13.5% are called *early adopters*. This is a group of people that are up-to-date on the latest trends and techniques within our profession. These same people always want to be first in line for whatever new product is on the market. These are the people that wait in line for the new iPhone just so they can be first. This group of people buy products because they see the vision of the 2.5% and it "clicks" with them immediately. Does this sound familiar to chiropractic patients? We often say, once a patient is treated and educated properly in chiropractic it seems to just "click" with them, and they love everything about chiropractic. They are the best patients because they are loyal, and they will always come to a chiropractor first with any health needs that they have. About 16% of the population are in the *innovators* and *early adopters* group, which hovers right around the percentage that the chiropractic profession has remained for so many years.

The next group is the *early majority* which is 34% of the entire market. Companies know that they must get their product to the mass market, and the *early majority* is the first group that they must reach for their product or service to be successful. However, there is what Everett Rodgers, the founder of this law, called *the Chasm*. The Chasm is what every product must cross before it can create mass appeal to that 34% of *early majority*. The way products cross that chasm is by opinions of trusted people in that early adopters group. This is why you see companies seeking celebrity endorsements because it causes a sense of confidence in a product if they see a face that they trust or to whom they are attracted. This group is also conscientious about the research regarding a product and are very skeptical until testimonials and research prove that this product will make their life better. If you can successfully cross *the Chasm* and reach that 34% of *early adopters*, you will have reached half the population with the 16% you had already reached.

The *late majority* is another 34% group and they will follow suit once the *early majority* has partaken in a product and it becomes clear that there is substantial benefit and is safe for them to use. If the product breaks into the first 34%, it is most likely to break into the second 34%, according to many sources.

The last 16% are *the laggards* who will not use any innovation and who prefer to stay with their comfortable lives as they know them. They still have dial up internet and push-button phones because they do not embrace change. Only few products make it into this group of the market as it is so hard to reach. The diffusion of innovation curve is supremely helpful, and we will see how the chiropractic profession can use this to its advantage.

You as a chiropractor have been stuck anywhere from 12-14% of the population of your city. Wouldn't you like to double that? There wouldn't be enough time in the day if you doubled your patient base. You might think that it is crazy to think that you could double your patient base within a year's time. You may be rational to think that, but according to the Law of Diffusion of Innovation, we are only 2-4% of the population away from crossing the chasm and breaking into the mass market of *early* and *late majority*. Think of the possibilities to our growth if we accomplished that. It is not going to happen just because we want it to, or because some practice management group says that their "tested and tried" formula will help you bring in more patients per month. We've all heard those pitches from Practice Management groups how easy it is if one just buys their $500 a month formula for success. All that these practice management groups are out to do is make money for themselves, not to push Chiropractic further in the market. This book differs in its methods because it seeks to display what we as chiropractors must do to raise the entire profession's outreach and reputation. No cost to you, just hard work and a lot of teamwork as a profession and these dreams will become realities.

Zero to One Thinking

Peter Thiel, co-inventor of PayPal, wrote a book titled *Zero to* One, which highlighted a new way of thinking about progress within an industry. He coined the term "Zero to One" to show that there is a better way to advance a product or an industry. He defines success in two different ways, horizontal progress and vertical progress. I am going to highlight both, and show how understanding this concept can benefit chiropractors as we seek to advance our profession.

Horizontal success was defined as *globalization*, or taking something that worked in one area and making it work everywhere around the world. Thiel used the example of a typewriter. If we take the basic design of a typewriter and mass produce it for the entire world to use, then we have made horizontal success. This is a very successful means of advancing cultures to new inventions but not a successful way at improving that typewriter. Many cultures have desired this technique of horizontal success by copying what the United States has used to become advanced. Thiel says China has been using this technique to copy everything that America did many years ago, to create growth within their economy. China's success can be attributed to horizontal success. They have not created anything new to introduce that America had not already done 50 years prior. This is the reason that China is seeing the success in their economy, because it is a "fool-proof" plan to boost its economy. This strategy is very helpful, but it is very limited.

Vertical success is defined as introducing *technology* into an already existing product or industry. Using the typewriter example, Thiel says that when Microsoft invented a word processor for the computer, it took a completely different path to success. No longer did someone follow the path that everyone else was doing-they decided something more needed to be done.

Technology, according to Webster, is defined as, "the application of scientific knowledge for practical purposes, especially in an industry." We see technology as something that revolves around computers, but that is not the essence of what that definition means. Technology is any method that improves the efficiency and proficiency of an already existing product. Every single major company in the United States has had to use technology to become the company they are today. Think of Amazon.com, Apple Inc., and the many others. No successful company has used horizontal success to become the company they are today. It must employ vertical success tactics.

Applying this concept to the chiropractic profession is not a difficult task. I want to pull back the sheets on chiropractors and show just where we must go and the changes we must make to change our future. We have been applying horizontal success to our profession for years. The way we do business is the major one. We have used our private-practice model since the inception of our profession. Every chiropractor has opened his practice's doors and hoped that patients would continue to come every month. Each chiropractor has his plan for how he can become successful within this model, and there have been many doctors that have used this model and created much success for themselves. These doctors thought much differently though than the rest of the chiropractors. They were entrepreneurs at heart, not physicians. They hired associates, opened multiple practices, and brought in other health care professionals to boost their individual profits. There is nothing wrong with this way of thinking, nor do I look down at these doctors for having an entrepreneurial mindset to their practice. These doctors are precisely the doctors that could have thought of this business model years ago, but they thought much too small. They thought about their practice, in their small city, and their reputation. They forgot that no matter how successful they were; that they were still chained to the entire profession. These doctors have accrued great success, but much more needs to be done for the entire profession.

The entire profession is not seeing the same success that these doctors are seeing in their practices. In school, I wondered why there were these successful doctors and also there was 30% of graduates that were not even in the profession after 5 years in practice. Is it because the profession did not provide every doctor with the opportunity to succeed? Chiropractic has tried to replicate its successes repeatedly, but now it has reached a critical mass. If nothing is done to change the current state of chiropractic, the entire profession will implode upon itself. This is the point that most industries sit down and think about what needs to be done to fix the problem. NOW is that time for Chiropractic.

Why is this proposed business model an example of vertical progress? It is vertical thinking because it is taking an old and broken system and finds a new way in which to do business. That is technology! Like Thiel said in "Zero to One", technology does not need to be new computers and gadgets; it is the process of making a system more efficient and more profitable. By implementing this technology into the profession, we will see that the profession can lift each doctor up and give him the success he dreamed of back in chiropractic school. The profession must begin to bring the doctors higher in success, rather than individual doctors trying to grunt and strain to pull the rest of the profession higher. We have had it backwards, and there must be a paradigm shift within the profession.

The age of individual success is over within chiropractic, though individual doctors will still be lauded for their successes and advances. This new business model is the largest idea to date within the profession, but it must be done before we reach that critical mass point. It is at that point, that all the successes that you have had will mean absolutely nothing. Everything we have accomplished in the last 100 years will mean nothing, if we sit on our hands as a profession.

The business of chiropractic must become the number one technological advance that we must pursue within the profession. Nothing will benefit us more than this. The beauty of this problem is that it has been identified, and the cure will be laid out. Now we must just act! It'll take a lot of work, but nothing great or necessary for success was ever easy.

Addition vs. Multiplication

We all grew up in grade school learning from our teachers the concepts of mathematics. No American child that I have known ever eluded a class in simple arithmetic. At first these numbers and signs all were very confusing to us, but after years and years of practice, these problems became much more manageable. I am not talking about geometry or calculus or any of the harder level mathematics, I exclusively want to talk about arithmetic in this chapter. You will see how these concepts of arithmetic can benefit us within the profession of chiropractic as we forge a new way of doing business.

Addition was probably the easiest problems that we ever encountered as children in grade school. 3+3=6. Nothing tricky about that, always straight forward and easy. As we became fluent in addition, the teachers would take us to subtraction where we soon mastered that concept as well. It wasn't until we got to multiplication that math class became a little bit harder. We saw 3x3 and instantly shouted out 6 because it looks so similar to the same problem that we saw a few months back, but with multiplication there is a much different outcome.

When addition and multiplication begin, there is some striking conclusions to be made. 1+1=2, but 1x1=1. Addition results in a higher outcome than multiplication does. Moving to 2+2=4, and 2x2=4 as well. Both addition and multiplication had the exact same outcome. It isn't until you move to the 3's that addition can no longer keep up with multiplication. 3+3=6, yet 3x3=9. As the numbers continue to grow, multiplication soon shows its superior dominance in reaching a higher outcome than addition. The interesting part is that at the beginning addition was actually a better strategy than multiplication (remember the 1's) for a greater outcome. Even with the 2's you could make the argument that addition was on par with multiplication. As time went on though you soon realized the restraints that addition had on it, and the freedom that multiplying had in arithmetic.

You may be reading this and say, "Oh my goodness did I seriously just get an arithmetic lesson from this guy?" And yes, you did, but it was integral in laying the groundwork for the thinking in chiropractic that I am going to share. When the private practice model was booming in all areas of healthcare, doctors of chiropractic were so quick to open their doors of service in any area they felt comfortable. This was extremely profitable too, as you could have been the only chiropractor for 30 miles. No competition led you to amazing profits and an extremely rewarding career. A few years later, a new doctor of chiropractic set up shop only 15 miles away from you. Things got a little more competitive as he took a few of your patients, but you weren't sweating too much as you still had so many patients to treat. This continued for a few years until another chiropractor caught wind of your city and moved his practice to within 10 miles of you. Competition was at an all-time high so you had to learn new techniques to continue to get new patients to come to your practice over the others. This paradigm continued for many years in chiropractic as a new chiropractor would come to town and try to start a practice in a city that was littered with every type of chiropractor that you could think of.

And that is where we are today in chiropractic. You cannot find any city of substantial population, where there isn't 1 chiropractor for every 400 people. Yet new graduates still go out and start new practices, thinking that they will be the successful ones in the area. This is foolish thinking, and it is also a detriment to the future of chiropractic. Competition is great, until competition becomes over-utilization. That means too many chiropractors and not enough patients, which is where we stand today.

The concept of addition was perfect for the start of chiropractic, as we all remember the glory days of chiropractic back in the 80's and 90's, but now we must look to multiplication instead of addition. Just like at the 1's and 2's, addition was great, but now we are trying to add 7+7 when we should be multiplying 7x7. Chiropractic has been around too long for us to continue to just open more solo doctor practices. We think that 7+7=14 is a good thing, but we have the opportunity to turn 14 into 49, if we just utilized multiplication.

Multiplying our practices together to create a supergroup or an IPA is the smartest thing to do as we need to pioneer new ways to get chiropractic into every home in the world. We know that what we have to offer is beneficial to everyone, yet we are trying to reach the world through adding more and more of the same type of practices. Only through sound business strategies can we have the capability to reach millions of more patients. I hope the example I used of arithmetic was helpful in showing the simplicity of this new concept. It is not that your practice is not successful in its current state, but what I am saying is that the chiropractic profession is not successful in its current state. Your practice can only go so high, because it is chained to the rest of the entire profession. If the profession refuses to grow, your business can only go as high as the ceiling provided. It's time we raise that ceiling within chiropractic, for everybody. This can be done, but we need to be willing to change our mindset from adding more and more of the same practices, to multiplying our practices together to fill a greater need.

3

Mass Market Permeability

Chiropractic has been stuck at 12% of the market for the past 30 years, and there are factors why the profession has plateaued at such an interesting percentage of the market. It is interesting especially after reading about the Law of Diffusion of Innovation. So many companies fail to cross the chasm and become confined to always reach only a small portion of the market. What makes the companies different that do cross into the mass market? I believe that there are four factors that our profession lacks that other industries and companies have.

The first factor is that the mass market just does not trust us yet to be effective in treatment. According to the Palmer Gallup study done on the "Perceptions of Chiropractic", 28% of people who have never been to a chiropractor thought that the chiropractic adjustment is extremely dangerous and 47% of people were uncertain or had no opinion. Those numbers are not good because it gives an average of a 40% approval rating for safety among those who have never been to a chiropractor before. That is worse than most President's approval ratings after they leave office. If we wonder why patients do not trust us to treat them properly, it can all stem from improper education. We can all agree that in the past the medical profession sought to discredit chiropractors, which may still happen, but there is a whole new generation of young people out there that are very open to alternative and holistic medicine. We must capture their attention before someone else diverts it from chiropractic's way of healing. This same study asked a question, "Would you talk to a chiropractor about general health, well-being, and nutrition?" Fifty-nine percent said that they disagree with ever talking to a chiropractor about those things. If that doesn't alarm you, I don't know what will! That is the aspect of health for which we are most effective. For almost 60% of responses to be negative is our fault as a profession. We cannot blame the Wilk's law suit against the AMA for these problems, as this shows a lack of effectiveness in communicating our message, and perhaps laziness on the profession to connect with the community and educate them on all the benefits we have to offer. The reason I think most chiropractors are unable to effectively communicate this message to the mass market is because that they are so busy trying to run their practice and juggle a personal life that they do not have enough time in the day to reach the public. It is a problem with our model of practice that inhibits this exposure, not a problem with our message. Once we realize that it is how we are running the profession that is the problem, only then can we effectively and efficiently fix this problem.

The second factor for not reaching mass market permeability is exactly what I stated in the last sentence of the previous paragraph. How we are running our profession is a major contributing factor to the plateau we see today. That is a very broad statement and may seem vague to most, so let me focus on what I mean. The business model we push in the profession is a solo practitioner model. According to the 2016 survey done by ChiroEconomics, 67% of chiropractors operate alone without the help of another D.C, M.D, or D.O. The majority of chiropractic businesses are one doctor trying to handle all the various conditions that come into his clinic without any outside help. This can be very daunting, especially for a chiropractor that may not feel completely confident with his knowledge in primary care. There has been a trend of late to go into group practice where multiple D.C.'s come together to form a practice which is a positive step, but it's still only at 30% of the practices. There are many chiropractors who are fortunate enough to work in an integrated healthcare setting, and have proven to do much better financially and have reduced responsibilities in this role. This has shown to be an effective model and shows that the more we come together with each other and with M.D.'s, the better off we are as a profession. We have now taken it to group practices where 2 or 3 D.C.'s come together, but what I will be proposing a model on a much larger scale.

The third factor in which our profession is run that is far too outdated is how we pursue diplomates and not residency programs. I believe the knowledge that we are getting in our diplomates is important and substantial enough to warrant some tremendous respect within the medical community. If you sit back and think about what the diplomate does for the practitioner, other than a knowledge-base in that course of study-you would be hard-pressed to find benefits in exclusivity to how they can practice. The 300 plus hours we put into our diplomate programs evolve our sense of how we want to practice, but the hours do not evolve our scope of practice. It is very important we understand that distinction.

If I wanted to get a diplomate in orthopedics, I would sign up for the program, pay my tuition, take the course and get my diplomate-this is all in hopes of creating a niche in the market for the skills that I have just received. If I were smart, I would then begin to network and market myself as a Chiropractic Orthopedist with advanced training in any injuries affecting the body, after all, that's what the diplomate taught me, but the Chiropractor across the street knew I was getting this diplomate and began to market himself heavily in the community and created a stronghold on the market while I finished my final exams. I would have just spent upwards of $5,000 for a piece of paper and some letters after my name with no patients or profit to show from it. This is a serious problem within our profession, and we need to protect the practice rights of those that decide to get advanced training in a specialty, similar to the medical profession. Though some practitioners have had tremendous growth after completing their diplomates, it would be nice if there were some exclusivity written into their scope of practice that allows them to be the only practitioners to treat such conditions.

If there were residency programs, this would funnel our profession's brightest minds into specialties for which they are passionate, while giving them exclusivity within the profession. This would not only give those practitioners an amazing advantage in the market, but also generate tremendous respect from our medical counterparts. The diplomate programs were well thought out by those running them, and they are seeing tremendous profits because they saw a hole in our education system and capitalized on it. Good for them, but now we must take our profession back and raise the standards for ourselves. This is a complex problem to fix, but with the proper business model that I am proposing, this hole in our education will be filled and will effectively works to enhance our profession.

The fourth and final factor our profession has not been able to break into the mass market is that we do not have the leadership required to lead our profession, inspire new advances, and effectively market chiropractic medicine. When B.J. Palmer was Chancellor of Palmer College of Chiropractic, he knew exactly what needed to be done to grow the profession, or as we call it, develop the profession. He earned the title, The Developer, because he increased the reach of chiropractic to the extent that we have it today. He inspired research at Palmer by devoting a premium of his time and money to his research facility. B.J. was ahead of his time integrating the use of X-ray technology that even his medical counterparts were slow to adopt. He increased the education requirements to a 3-year program and he motivated chiropractors all around the world with his drive to better the profession. With his death in 1961, we lost the greatest component to what Chiropractic is today. Looking at the advances he made in his lifetime and comparing them to where we are now, our profession that has not decided to push further and strive for more.

What have we done in the last 50 years that B.J didn't already do? We still use the safety pin analogy, B.J. started that. We hold fast to the theory of subluxation without trying to innovate ways in which to quantify or substantiate our claims. Staying true to our roots as a profession is fine, but we must innovate past what they did in the early 1900's to grow. This is not any one person's fault, but it does cast a dark shadow as to where we are in 2017. As a profession, we know the art and philosophy, now let's substantiate the science of our amazing healing art. This can be done by having a unified approach to running our industry. We are an entire industry, not a bunch of individuals trying to survive on our own. **We need to act like an industry and become unified.** That happens when someone or a group of people step forward and decide that they want more. I know I want more, and that's why I am writing this book and laying out my vision. I want chiropractic to change the lives of everyone on this planet. For those that understand and agree with what I am saying, step up in your community. Whether that means getting all the chiropractors in your city and deciding how to innovate the market, coming together as a state and finding ways to communicate this vision across the state, or unifying as a profession across the nation and following a vision for each of us to follow, we must have leaders who sacrifice their lives to better us all.

Identifying problems and fixing them are two completely different processes. I've tried to identify them as best as I know, but we cannot be complacent anymore. There must be a hunger for more in every one reading this, or else you wouldn't have continued to read this book. Building an industry will not be easy; there will be setbacks and failures along the way, but if we can enrich the lives of our patients and create a better future for those coming behind us; I think we will look back and see the grand success of it all.

What can you do to fix these problems? After all one chiro cannot carry this model alone? Nothing could be farther from the truth. Each chiropractor has a unique responsibility to now project this vision and message to the rest of the colleagues around them. Give them this book and let them catch the dream for themselves. We must inspire those around us if we want them to follow wholeheartedly. No one else in your community is thinking of doing such a transcendent action right now. They are just trying to figure out how to pay their bills when it comes to the first of the month. This gives a leading edge, each chiropractor who wants this model must position yourself as the expert in their community on how every chiropractor can grow. This is a huge undertaking and shouldn't be tackled alone. Those who want this needed change in their community can always consult with myself and other experts in other fields as to how to pursue the dreams to create the largest chiropractic center in the world, equipped with the newest research and development, groundbreaking residencies, and substantial profits.

4

Unity, R&D, Residencies

Apple, Inc. has had success that few companies in the course of human history have ever seen. With Steve Jobs at the helm of this company, it soared to its position as the leading technology company today. Steve Jobs accomplished this with passion for his product, developing that product, and educating his employees on the vision he had. Taking a page out of his playbook and converting it into our profession, we too can surge chiropractic to the forefront of the medical community as the leader in the healthcare industry. One of my favorite quotes from Jobs himself is, "My model for business is the Beatles. They were four guys who kept each other's kind of negative tendencies in check. They balanced each other, and the total was greater than the sum of the parts. That's how I see business: great things in business are never done by one person, they're done by a team of people." We are a family of chiropractors, and we all have our quirks and idiosyncrasies, but we need each other, and we must unite ourselves to pursue these three pillars to our success.

The first pillar to success must be that of Unity. Andrew Carnegie once said, "Teamwork is the ability to work together toward a common vision. The ability to direct individual accomplishments toward organization objectives. It is the fuel that allows common people to attain uncommon results." If a patient with an injury went to 15 chiropractors, he would get 15 different ways to fix his problem. This is true because we each have our own creative mindset, guided by our different techniques and solidified by our anecdotal evidence that has worked on previous patients. If that same patient told one chiropractor the opinion of the previous chiropractor, that physician would most likely diminish the credibility and value of the other doctor's technique and philosophy. The profession has done a disservice to this patient as he is confused who is right and what is his problem. This occurs every day across America, and it destroys our profession each time it happens.

Why does this situation happen in the first place? More often than not, each chiropractor is out to make his own money and advance his practice even if that means diminishing his colleague across the street. That chiropractor may not know if the other doctor's technique would be successful; but because it is different, it must be wrong. We all have our favorite techniques that we love, whether it's Gonstead, Diversified, Palmer Package, Upper Cervical, or a host of other options.

Which one is the best? They all seem to work when utilized by the properly trained professional.

If a patient were treated upper cervical on his Co/C1, Gonstead on his lumbar spine, and Functional Neurology applied to balance his nervous system, the possibilities for success would be unparalleled. However, these techniques will never come together for the simple reason that the professionals refuse to admit that they cannot fix everything. NO technique can fix every problem that walks through the door, yet there would be no way we would consider referring every headache patient to the upper cervical doctor across town. We would lose so much of our business, even if we were unable to properly treat it with our technique's training. Why did we create a climate where intra-professional referrals are so rare? The answer is that our industry's business model is flawed. The model I will propose effectively lays out a system where these practitioners can make these intra-professional referrals within the same business structure without hurting their bottom lines. How can we fix this problem within chiropractic? First, we must understand our technique's shortcomings and applaud the successes of the other techniques.

Super Bowl XLIX was nothing short of an amazing example of how applauding the successes of others can lead to greater unity and future successes. The shock factor of the Malcolm Butler interception of Russel Wilson at the 1-yard line is a memory that will live forever in the moments of Super Bowl history. The Patriots won their fourth Super Bowl, and Tom Brady was crowned MVP of the game. Brady had all but clenched his title as the greatest quarterback of all time after this win with his MVP performance. As part of the rewards of winning MVP, he received a brand new red 2015 Chevy Silverado. Tom Brady could have taken that new truck and enjoyed his successes and all the accolades for himself, but instead he made an unprecedented move that paid off in a big way. Brady gave the MVP truck to Malcolm Butler, who in his mind, was the true MVP of the game. Brady realized that his success was due to the performance of Butler, and he could not have done it without him. It was a great show of respect and appreciation for the work that someone else did for the overall team success. With this move by Brady, the Patriot's unity became stronger, and they would eventually go on to win another Super Bowl just two years later. Why is this story significant to us as Chiropractors? We can learn that appreciating the successes of another chiropractor in turn benefits us. We are all on the same team, if we adopt this Brady character trait across the profession and truly recognize what others are accomplishing, our profession moves forward together to accomplish more. If Tom Brady had not given the credit to Malcolm Butler would they have won that championship two years later. I don't think so and here's why. Who would have wanted to play for a team where a quarterback was all about himself? The Patriots would not have been able to grow their team with talent if all the free agents would have known that if they did a good job on the field, Tom Brady would get all the credit. The same goes for our profession; we must applaud and pronounce the successes of other techniques or practitioners. Though this seems counter-intuitive to business, it will lift the profession as a whole. This could be realized if we had a business model within the profession where the successes of all techniques were allowed to benefit the whole and not just the individual.

The second pillar of success that our profession should focus on is the advancement of research & development (R&D) for the profession. New technologies come out every year from companies like Apple and Microsoft. They have entire divisions of their companies set up for R&D. These divisions are not put on the backburner while they try to force iPhones down consumer's throats. No, they are at the forefront of their focus and funding. It is in this division where new technologies are supplied to the market and advancement of human culture are experienced.

Why are there no Research & Development Divisions in chiropractic? I heard of a small scholarship awarded to any student that goes above and beyond and finishes some research while in school. I also know of Christine Goertz D.C. and her amazing research she is pumping into the profession, but why aren't her efforts and accomplishments the norm for our profession? We place a premium on practicing clinicians and not on the researchers and developers of new technology for our profession. Many graduates from a chiropractic school will set off into the realm of starting their own practice or working for someone else's practice, but when comes the innovation? The problem is we do not value or put funding into R&D for the profession. No single aspect will drive the profession farther into the future than this concept.

Systematically, we could evaluate students while in school and give them real careers and passions for research of a technique or other important science that must be validated through peer-reviewed research. Also, we could find the brilliant minds in the profession who would rather innovate new technologies than muddle around for their lives treating patients that they may not fully enjoy. We could give incentives to these people, and in return, we would have an influx of new ideas and research to grow the profession. We could successfully do this in a unified model, but with the current state of chiropractic, these geniuses within the profession will never have the opportunity to create a breakthrough. There may be a chiropractic innovators but they are stuck working a 9-5 job that is preventing you from an idea they have formulated. This book can provide you with the hope that our profession is on the right path to giving chiropractors the opportunity to have their research or innovation the funding and attention that it needs to become reality.

The third and final pillar of success that our profession needs to pursue is that of residency programs. I have touched on this issue before because it is extremely vital to our success as a profession in the future. Today's medical climate calls for specialized professionals to help with a wide variety of complex medical issues. With people suffering from so many life-style related conditions, chiropractors are well-suited for success in the future. The time is now to provide an extensive residency to our degrees. This will provide the healthcare field with professionals who are well-trained and will provide patients with doctors who are holistic in mindset and protect them from medications that could do more harm than good. These residencies will create exclusivity to certain protocols and techniques just like a residency within the medical model does. A cardiac surgeon is an expert in cardiothoracic surgery, so if an ACL tear comes into his practice he makes the proper referral to an orthopedic surgeon. He does not try to treat this patient with all the skills he learned back in medical school to help this patient, but he realizes his limitations in helping this patient and allows someone else to care for the patient. In the chiropractic profession, we see doctors that have diplomates in many fields and call themselves experts, yet they try to treat patients out of their specialty all the time, with substandard results. This goes on every day in the profession. While the practitioner down the road took a diplomate in neurology and would be able to help that patient with superior results, but that patient went to a chiropractor who likes focuses on soft tissue pathologies. Though we know there is some cross-over in the profession, we should be able to make those referrals without worrying about our bottom lines. These residencies will also allow doctors who have pursued an extensive residency certain exclusivities in their scope of practice. This protects those doctors, and will also motivate each chiropractor to find their passion and niche within the market. The last benefit to residency programs is the validation of our education within the medical community. We need to show our dedication to life-long education and patient care. More referrals would come from hospitals and medical doctors if they were 100% confident that the chiropractor was absolutely capable of treating their patient. These programs haven't been implemented because of the current model in which we do business. There is not the ability to have residents at your local chiropractic practice; but if a system were set up within the new unified chiropractic model, this would allow for residency programs in a vast array of specialties.

5

The Change:

Unified Chiropractic Model

The Unified Chiropractic Model is the sole-reason why this book was written. No other business model within the healthcare profession has been proposed for chiropractors to use, that will guarantee this amount of unity and profitability for the entire profession. As I delve into the inter-workings of this plan, try to imagine yourself, in your city, using this model to enhance the access of chiropractic to thousands more people.

The Unified Chiropractic Model seeks to bring every chiropractic physician of all different techniques and philosophies into one centralized clinic, for the purpose of better communication between chiropractors, to create better outcomes for patients. This unity is so important because when patients come into these clinics, there can be a coalition of doctors and residents that can generate treatment plans tailored specifically for their case, which increases the probability of them having a resolution of symptoms. This has never been an option in chiropractic before because we are a splintered profession, but imagine the brightest minds in every specialty in our profession working together to get patients better. Unfortunately, all chiropractors are out to pursue their own dreams of how to deliver care in their offices.

We must create a standard of care for the entire profession, with regards to every treatment that we do in chiropractic. Instead of one doctor of chiropractic working in an office, the unified chiropractic model seeks to bring 15+ doctors of chiropractic together in a city. This clinic will be in the center of town where thousands of people drive by each day and will have the newest and most researched technologies our profession has to offer. These clinics will provide doctors of chiropractic all the tools necessary to diagnose and treat any patients that seeks chiropractic care.

As we transition into these new facilities, we will maintain the same atmosphere that every small chiropractic office had in them before. We must make our patients feel like the most important people in the world, who are receiving our undivided attention. That is the one quality our profession does so well, and we cannot let that aspect leave, even though we are stepping into state of the art facilities. I am convinced that when clinics of this magnitude are being raised, they will draw so much attention from their communities, that we will be able to reach so many more people with the amazing potential that chiropractic could have for their health. This generated interest within the communities will be capitalized on by our entire team as we seek to generate interest in demographics that have never considered going to a chiropractor before. Currently, chiropractors do not have the time or the energy to reach out into their communities because they are so busy trying to run their own practice. With a unified model, we will now have the personnel to reach into those communities and begin conversations with groups of people that never have considered chiropractic care before. That has never been a reality before in chiropractic, but now it will be the norm for our clinics to sponsor area sports teams, sponsor health and wellness fairs, and also get more involved in community events in each of these cities. This will allow more people to have exposure to the great things our profession has to offer to their lives.

The Unified Chiropractic Model will also create economies of scale that will allow us to save more money each year on overhead, and also generate more and more income every year as we increase our patient base. The ways we will reduce overhead in each of these centers are: by reducing the amount of employees, reducing rent and equipment, and by creating efficient systems of management. We will not require large amounts of front desk, chiropractic assistants, and other staffers that frequently are hired by every office. We will only hire the best staff from each of the clinics already in the community, so that we have a smooth transition into the new facility with the best possible staff already familiar with chiropractic offices. Not only can we save on payroll, but also begin to spend much less on overhead with regards to paying for rent, utilities, and equipment needed to run these centers. Though these clinics will be the largest centers to date within the profession, they will dramatically reduce excessive waste within the profession. Specific details of reducing overhead will vary depending on every locations, however, the general concept of reducing overhead in these clinics while increasing the standard of care will be a top priority.

Imagine a city of 150,000 people with around 20 different chiropractors fighting over the 12% of those people that are already chiropractic patients. Practices are stretched thin, and chiropractors are over-worked trying to treat existing patients, while attracting new ones each month. This creates so much burn-out with each of these doctors and practices because they never get vacation time, nor do they have an abundance of money to afford closing down the clinic for a few weeks. Our profession has created doctors that are facing both burn-out and bankruptcy all because our model of doing business is severely flawed.

However, within the Unified Chiropractic Model, each of these chiropractors will work together as a team to increase patient care and increase profits for their center. With 15 or more doctors in each facility, this will allow doctors to enjoy vacation time, without fear of dramatically losing business while away. Another benefit will be that each doctor will be able to get back to being a doctor again. In the current state of chiropractic, the doctor is the business owner first, then chiropractor. This takes him away from treating patients to worrying about cleaning toilets, doing payroll, and fixing broken appliances. In this unified center, the doctors can focus on getting their patients better and leave the business and the mundane tasks of running a business to less occupied minds.

I have to stop and address one thing to each of you doctors that are considering yourself in this position. You may be asking yourself, why in the world would I become an employee of a new clinic, when I am the boss and owner at my current one?

Each of the doctors that choose to come into these new facilities built by The D.C Initiative, will be part-owners and board members of their respected clinics. Having doctors run these centers, will be a tremendous benefit to our centers because now each decision that is made by the board is made by doctors who are concerned about patient care first, and profits second. This creates a stark difference between our centers and hospitals. I do not want business men and CEO's telling our doctors and staff how to treat patients because it will make the business more money. I want every decision made at these centers to be by doctors who know exactly what is best for our patients, and not our pocketbooks. This is not to say that each doctor will not make more money each year. Studies have shown that when doctors come together, each doctor's salary and quality of life drastically increases.

The team here at The D.C Initiative is committed to getting these spectacular centers built in cities all across the world. I lay out a detailed step-by-step plan in a later chapter of how we go from multiple clinics in a city to having one centralized chiropractic clinic. The details of different contracts, permits, and business loans will all be handled by The D.C Initiative, which will allow you as the doctors to continue to practice and make money at your practice, while we construct the new facility utilizing the Unified Chiropractic Model.

6

Implementing the Change

"Do not confuse motion and progress. A rocking horse keeps moving but does not make any progress."-Alfred A. Montapert

Speaking about these problems is exactly what we have been doing within the profession for so many years. Just like the rocking horse, what have we accomplished through these discussions? We must finally do something about it and create progress; yes, CREATE progress. The steps to accomplish this overhaul of the profession begins with one person in a community that wants more in his career. The challenges that our profession faces today are immense and I recognize that, but we must put in the work today to avoid these consequences if left untreated.

"By failing to prepare, you are preparing to fail."-Benjamin Franklin

Franklin's quote has been used by many to motivate people to properly plan-out exactly how they are going to accomplish something in life. This could be used by a professional athlete, as he must put tremendous time and energy into his skill before he can compete against other professional athletes. It also can be used for businesses and how they must strategically plan how they are going to create their business to make it successful. No business ever gets created without a business plan, or at least a well-thought out idea of how to run their company. No one ever just makes it out of blind luck in the business world, and neither will we. Dwight D. Eisenhower said it best, "Luck is where preparation meets opportunity." To make this business model work for the chiropractic profession, we must have a plan. What this chapter entails are the day-to-day plans how we can effectively and efficiently bring a city of chiropractors together in our unified chiropractic model.

Step 1: Initial meetings to determine goals and to create a list of potential members

After contacting The D.C Initiative, a meeting date will be set with all the chiropractors in the city of interest. In these meetings, plans will be shown to all the chiropractors about the potential for their city and how it could benefit them individually. If there continues to be interest once the presentation has finished, then a list of potential members will be drafted. As the group begins to form, open discussion about the short and long-term goals from each member will be recorded, so that each party can have input into how the business will run and operate.

Step 2: Draft a letter of intent and members will sign a confidentiality agreement.

Each member must sign a letter of intent, so that the group knows it can count on the support from its members throughout the entire process. The confidentiality agreement is meant to protect the business model from being copied by an opposing party after the meeting is over. All this should be done soon after that initial meeting. The confidentiality agreement will be signed by every doctor that attends the conference.

Step 3: Form a Limited Liability Company and obtain a new federal tax identification number.

The steps to forming the framework for how this new practice will run will be determined in these steps. A supergroup is the desired form of business, but that must be agreed upon before this step can be finalized. Examples of the different forms of businesses will be explained in later chapters.

Step 4: Forming an Executive Committee

The executive committee's purpose will be to hold weekly meetings ironing out the details how the merger of this practice will work. Also, financial documents will be obtained by every practice desiring to be a part of the group. This will help the executive committee to organize detailed projections on the size and success of the practice. The executive committee will be made up of voted members from the group of potential chiropractors.

Step 5: Analyze financial and legal information from prospective chiropractors

This step is one of the most important because it will give the executive committee insight into the potential financials of the practice once it is fully formed. Also, knowing the assets that each practice can donate to the group is important in determining the value and ownership that each practice will have within the group. The value of each individual practice in the group will be laid out in a future chapter.

Step 6: Prepare operational and organizational agreements.

These agreements will highlight how the practice will be run, how the management and ownership will be delegated, and will lay a basic-foundation to the financial compensation for each owner/chiropractor in the practice.

Step 7: Evaluate any legal issues with regards to how the group is set up

This will be carried out by an attorney who specializes in healthcare law and anti-trust law, so the group will ensure that no laws are broken in the formation of this group. This is important in a healthcare setting, since there are laws regarding "price-fixing" in a city. Price fixing is when doctors from a city get together to determine an amount that they will all charge for their services. This will be avoided by carefully forming the structure of this practice to ensure that no wrong-doing has occurred.

Step 8: Forming Care Center agreements

Forming standard of care agreements and daily operations documents will be paramount to the success of this practice. The group will only run on systems that are set in place for how patient care will be handled. This must be agreed upon by each doctor, not just the executive committee.

Step 9: Forming a Board of Directors

This board is different from the executive committee, though it could hold the same members. This Board is responsible for the business of the practice. Weekly meetings by this board to discuss reports and other documents to ensure the success of the practice. The Board of Directors will be voted by the entire group.

Step 10: Create policies and procedures to ensure legal compliance (billing and HIPAA compliance)

This step will be completed by the Board of Directors and will establish the systems that will determine how the practice will be run.

Step 11: Pursue vendor contracts

This will include but will not be limited to: practice location (building or leasing), EHR contracts, equipment contracts, vendor contracts, etc.

Step 12: Negotiate banking agreements

Proper amounts of capital needed for the center will be determined and investors will be sought after to fund the project. Completed by Board of Directors.

Step 13: Hire appropriate staff

Determining the needs of the practice, and filling them with experienced personnel. Many employees from the doctor's former practices will be hired to fill desired roles.

Step 14: Establish "Launch Date"

The Board will establish a launch date, and will complete the movement of each practice into the new location. Heavy marketing will be done throughout this process to inform existing patients and the public about the new location.

Step 15: Prepare for Grand Opening

The time frame from Step 1-15 should take about one year, if done efficiently. Proper planning is to be done through each of these steps in preparation for day 1. Though one year is the goal, each step must be met before the doors can be opened. This practice's success is determined on the careful planning of each member of this group.

These steps have been proven successful in the formation of many medical group practices over the last few years. Many medical doctors have run into the same problems that current chiropractors are facing, but they found a way to combat these problems by coming together. This forms unity within the profession and will form a direction in which the profession can grow towards. This group will be the first of its kind within the chiropractic profession and will become the foundation to how chiropractors do business in the future.

7

Options for Business Structure

There are different options how this group can operate. In those early steps of implementation, these different options must be weighed as to which option is best for the entire group. The options are between a <u>Supergroup</u> or an <u>Independent Practice Associations (IPA)</u>.

First, a Supergroup is a collection of initially separate practices, joining a single entity or group to achieve specific advantages.

The advantages to forming a supergroup are as follows:

1. Reduce overhead expense

This is accomplished by hiring one staff for the entire group. Many chiropractors have hired multiple employees to run their private practice, but once a group is formed the staff can be shared. This can be from front staff attendants, insurance billers, and chiropractic assistants. Having one staff for the entire group, reduces costs tremendously and creates higher efficiency in the center. When there is one properly trained staff, each member can fill his/her role to the betterment of the team. Another way overhead is trimmed is by sharing the expense of the building. Using one centralized location to conduct business is more efficient and more cost-effective. With the extra funds from joining forces, the group can also be located in a more attractive and larger building, and perhaps in a better location in the city, which will attract more new patients. Other ways that overhead can be cut is by sharing equipment and other office supplies. These monthly expenses can be quite costly for an individual doctor, but when a group is involved these expenses become less burdensome on the financial success of the practice.

2. Provide insurance for the entire group of physicians

By purchasing insurance for the entire group of physicians, this also creates a better policy for each physician while lowering the cost that it takes to cover that doctor. Though chiropractic insurance is historically very low, it can also be a way to reduce overhead expenses.

3. Gain leverage in managed care contracts

This is a huge benefit to a group of chiropractors working together. Each individual chiropractor negotiates his contracts with insurance companies and does not have much of an option to negotiate the terms of that contract. He must accept that contract and what the insurance company will pay him or else be limited to which patients he can treat. As a city of chiropractors, it would be illegal for the doctors to negotiate as one voice in their contracts, as that would violate "anti-trust" restrictions. The formation of this supergroup of chiropractors would give leverage in negotiating better terms for their services as chiropractors. This would provide better reimbursement rates for the services provided in this group. Insurance companies prefer working with groups of doctors, as opposed to multiple private practice doctors, so everyone wins.

4. Invest in future growth

Many chiropractors rarely have enough money at the end of the month to funnel back into the practice for future growth. This is solely because their expenses are far too great and their profits are too small. When a profitable business model is introduced into this supergroup, profits can then be used wisely to effectively grow the practice through each of the phases mentioned in a future chapter.

The disadvantages to forming a supergroup are as follows:

1. Individual doctor losing appearance of autonomy

Each doctor loves the idea of owning his own practice one day, and would initially avoid the idea of not having his own business to run. This could be a downside to forming a supergroup since each doctor would form under the new business tax identification number and would conduct business and billing under the new business number.

2. Hiring and Firing Staff

Trimming overhead means having to release unneeded staff members of previous practices and hiring only those that are necessary to the success of the group. This can be an awkward and painful step for many doctors, but this step can be accomplished by the board of directors. Each previous employee can apply for positions at the new practice, but would need to go through the same interview process as everyone else.

These two disadvantages can either be looked at as a blessing or as a roadblock for some doctors. They both can be a blessing, as it is a result of a more efficient and profitable business model for chiropractic. If doctors cannot agree on forming a supergroup, then an Independent Practice Association can be considered.

An Independent Practice Association (IPA) is basically a "practice without walls." This means that each practice retains their autonomy while sharing the same building as multiple other clinics.

The advantages to forming an IPA are as follows:

1. Sharing of expenses, such as leasing of building and equipment.
2. Each doctor would retain his autonomy and have full control over his patient's care.

Some disadvantages to forming an IPA compared to a supergroup are as follows:

1. More staff per doctor would need to be hired, as each physician would retain his private practice in the new building.
2. Difficulty in coordination amongst different practices. This would make it hard for each practice to communicate and would hinder the growth of chiropractic into a broader patient base.

Understandably these different options have their advantages and disadvantages. The D.C Initiative is fond of the supergroup because of the larger amounts saved in overhead, while communication among the entire profession is greater under one unified group. Though both models have been proven to be effective and more cost-effective than multiple private practices, the supergroup offers more benefits to the future of chiropractic.

This endeavor will start like a group practice, but once proper systems and techniques are implemented into the structure of the business, the different departments in the center will begin to take shape. As I mention later, there are specific phases to the proper steps for growth. This project cannot be done all at once; it is too expensive for that, but if we build a sustainable model, then the financing for the larger dreams will become a reality. One area where change will occur is in the marketing and advertising aspect of the practice. When one is by himself as a chiropractor he does not have much money to spend on marketing. This is one of the main reasons why his practice has not grown to date. When we have a marketing budget in the thousands of dollars per month, proper growth will be evidenced. Not only will the marketing budget increase but also our referrals from lawyers and medical doctors. Networking will be done by The D.C Initiative to area lawyers and medical doctors to explain the change in trajectory that the city chiropractors are taking. The lawyers will want to send their personal injury cases to our clinic as we will provide the best care for them-and will get them back to maximum medical improvement (MMI) much more quickly. Not only the lawyers, but also the medical doctors will begin referring patients more frequently. With a united chiropractic front in the city, medical doctors will feel much more comfortable sending their patients to our practice when they know they are getting the best care available. This will in turn skyrocket the percentage of patients that we see at our clinic.

I also want to add that patients who have contemplated chiropractic care before will now be more willing to try it because of the new facility being constructed, and also they will feel as if everyone is now using chiropractic care for a better life. I project that just by setting up this unified chiropractic center the percentage of patients will double within a year's time. Theses chiropractic centers would be one of the leading medical facilities in a given city, which would be a big change from what it is currently. **There are big steps between the current state of chiropractic in each city and what it could be, but it must begin with one person taking the initiative to sacrifice his comfort for the benefit of the entire profession.**

As mentioned in the different phases, it cannot begin with all 7 departments running from day one. Instead building a core group of general chiropractors working together to maximize patient outcomes, increase rate of patients within the community visiting our chiropractors; and thus, seeing a dramatic increase in the profits of chiropractic. There is a definite strategy to building these centers, and if followed properly, it will result in the largest and most successful chiropractic centers in the world.

Once a group practice across a city has been established, it will look very similar to a large group practice. Each chiropractor will continue to see patients that he did in his former clinic. No one will lose patients or have their patients given to another provider. The big difference in how this model works at first is that each doctor will share a staff and share the cost of overhead. I will get into how much a typical city of chiropractors is spending each month and how much they could save just by forming this group effort. As mentioned, this will show to be heavily profitable for the doctors as they do less work and make more money. As the percentage of patients increases and as the needs arise, hiring of specialty doctors will commence. A priority will be placed on those specialties that are the most needed in your specific demographic. If there is a large sports community, then a doctor with a Diplomate of the American Chiropractic Board of Sports Physicians (DACBSP) will be hired to meet the imposed demands. If there were a large number of patients with neurological conditions, then professionals such as Fellow of the American College of Functional Neurology (FACFN) and/or a Fellow of the International Academy of Clinical Neurology (FIACN) will be hired to help treat the demands of patients. As we continue to grow our patient base these specialists will be required to join our growing practice. Once these professionals have been hired, then the Departments can begin to take shape within the practice. One can begin to see the basic framework for how this practice could grow from just a regular group practice to a large institution when all hands are on deck, and a sound business strategy is in place.

8

Phases of Growth

"Everyone wants to live on top of the mountain, but all the happiness and growth occurs while you're climbing."-Andy Rooney

Throughout this book, I have discussed how the chiropractic profession must grow and move towards new goals. Growth is a very important word in business, so that is why I have dedicated an entire chapter to the phases for growth of this venture.

I have a certain philosophy about growth that bleeds into this idea of mine. I believe solely in *organic growth*. Many may know what that means, but if you don't, I will try to explain it in a few ways. Organic growth is much different from its counterpart which I call, *manufactured growth*. Organic growth is when a company begins as a small start-up and if the business is run efficiently will be able to slowly grow into a giant in about 10-15 years. Manufactured growth is when a company with a great idea, presents an idea to venture capitalists or angel investor and asks for millions of dollars for their business idea, in hopes of exploding into a giant company overnight.

This technique is done repeatedly in Silicon Valley, with the likes of Twitter, Snapchat, and even Tesla. What is one thing each of these companies all have in common? Each of these monster companies has never made a profit. How could Twitter or Snapchat never make money, when there are so many people that use these products? These companies create revenue, but they have not created profits for their shareholders yet, and may never. This is because each of these companies grew so quickly and borrowed so much money to get started that their growth has not been able to exceed the cost of starting up and the cost of running their businesses. Even Elon Musk has not been able to generate a profit at Tesla with his electric luxury cars. Surely someone as intelligent as Elon Musk could fix those problems at Tesla Motors, but even Tesla cannot break even and create profits for shareholders. Now Tesla will make a profit eventually, but they are going to have to get very business savvy in the process. They are going up against industry strongholds like Ford, GM, and Mercedes. Each of these companies organically grew over decades of time and now are poised to price Tesla out of the market. Each of these companies proved over a long period that they could make a profit. Now with Tesla coming onto the scene with their electric motor, these giant companies are seeing a market that wasn't there before. The good thing for companies like Ford, GM, and Mercedes is that they can now invest billions of their own money into an electric line of vehicles, that will price Tesla out of the market. As these companies continue to make profit with their internal combustion engine vehicles, they can make electric cars that are more affordable to the public, which will force Tesla to change a lot about their current course of action. I like Tesla, Snapchat, and Twitter; I just know that organic growth is more promising for the future because you are then entrenched in an industry. **In the game of quick start-ups and quick profits, there is never a promise of tomorrow.**

Chiropractic could use the same strategies that Tesla, Twitter, and Snapchat used and seek venture capital to fund this huge idea, and someone out there may just lend the money, but just like these other companies, we will be fighting for years to ever break even, though there would be increased revenues. For these reasons, I propose a growth strategy like that of Henry Ford's automotive company. He took a luxury item (the automobile), and made a process (assembly line) and used business techniques to get the car into the homes of Americans across this country. He organically grew his business into what it is today, a giant in the automotive industry. Chiropractic is just like the automobile 1900. Some people have access to chiropractic (12%), but we must use strategies to get chiropractic into the lives of every American. That is what this business model will do. It allows an environment for chiropractic to finally be successful for every chiropractor of this generation and for many generations to come. As these large chiropractic centers begin to pop up all over the nation, we will see that organic growth within the profession that we so desperately need right now.

Every business needs growth to survive and chiropractic is no different. We can manufacture growth within the profession, and make it look like we are successful, or we can follow these **phases of growth** to grow organically and build a prosperous future for all chiropractors for years to come.

Phase 1:

A large number of chiropractic physicians will come together to form a group business model that can focus on increase patient care and increase profitability. Each of them will be hired because they are already a part of this community. They will fulfil the needs of that practice since they have the base patient market of 12% that this practice will need to grow. As each chiropractor shares the expenses, the responsibility of running the business, and the patient care load; profits will soon begin to rise quite dramatically within the business. Doctors will be making more money because less staff is needed to run the practice, the cost of rent and utilities will be lower as the practice will be minimized to one large facility, instead of 15 mediocre facilities. Marketing budgets will be brought together to properly fund efforts to reach a broader patient base. All this is possible just by forming a large group practice with willing chiropractors in a city. What about the chiropractors who do not want to be a part of the group? Won't they be the competition? Yes, initially they will fight to take a portion of that 12% of the patients, but put yourself in the shoes of the patients. Would you rather go to the group of doctors in the new building, with all the newest equipment, or to the chiropractor that is in the strip mall next to a Chinese restaurant? This group practice will eventually overtake the existing market because we will bring more value to patients.

Another issue is larger cities that are too big for one centralized location. After all, patients do not want to drive more than 10 miles to get to their doctor. We can strategically place two or three practices within cities with that issue, but it would all be under one name so patients would know to go to our centers across the city if they want the best care. Our business would then begin to thrive financially once we all work together. The responsibilities of running the business would be upon a CEO and a board of doctors. The CEO could be a chiropractor or any person the board sees fit to run the company. The board of doctors would be filled with each of the doctors who helped start the center. This will give them input into how they want their practice to run, without the daily stress of running the business. All these steps will create profits that allow for phase 2 of the overhaul of our profession.

Phase 2:

Once the group practice has been formulated based on the existing chiropractors in that city, steps to specialize the practice will then become the next goal of the practice. The group of chiropractors who have started the practice will form the General Chiropractic Department. They will treat any typical chiropractic case that comes into the office. The specialist who will be recruited will become the Head Physicians in their department. Those specialists will be doctors who have received diplomates in Functional and Clinical Neurology, Pediatrics, Geriatrics, Sports & Rehabilitation and Radiology. Each of these doctors will be experts in their fields with years of experience with patient care. The patients we will funnel to their departments will be out of the group of patients that we have been able to build in Phase 1. If a patient under the age of 13 comes into the practice, then they would be treated in the Pediatric Department; a patient with a neurological disorder would be treated in the Neurology department. Each department will then start with a base of patients that have already been within the practice and continue to grow from that point. As patients come into the practice, they will first be seen by a General Chiropractor; and if the patient presents with a specific condition or special circumstance ,then they would be referred to the proper department. This will create intra-professional referrals and increase communication with chiropractors who have different techniques or specialties. As the base of patients continues to grow within these specialties, targeted marketing would then be employed to inform patients and medical professionals of the new opportunities of care at our center. As we educate patients and medical doctors on what we can accomplish, there will be an increase of value, interest, and utilization of these centers. All of this will happen while increasing profits and strengthening the reputation of the doctors at your center. Once the center is thriving, then Phase 3 can begin.

Phase 3:

Phase 3 is about the future of chiropractic, which entails the formation of residency programs in each of our departments and a fully operational research and development facility within the center. The residencies would change based on chiropractic school involvement in our facilities, but they will be utilized to further validate the education of Doctor of Chiropractic and increase the exposure of chiropractic students to specialized education in the areas of their interests. This will be beneficial to each center because the residents would then take some of the responsibility of patient care away from the head physicians which would allow those doctors to train the residents on proper utilization of chiropractic. This will give the chiropractic profession a group of residents that have been trained at these state-of-the-art centers to be the best doctors our profession can offer. This will increase the reputation of each center across the United States and around the world, which will result in a broader outreach and impact that chiropractic can have on patients.

The second step to Phase 3 is the implementation of a fully functional Research and Development (R&D) facility. In previous chapters, I have displayed the reasons that this is important to our profession, and now I will show why it is beneficial to these new centers. Having this unified business model will allow our head researcher easy access to large amounts of data that he can compile and formulate into research. This will create a pipeline of research coming out of each center, which benefits the entire profession. Imagine the amounts of research that can be done when all patient care is done under one roof and EHR system. This will allow studies to be done within the community to validate the claims of chiropractic. The researchers can apply for NIH grants and other loans to fund his research, but we must create an environment where he/she can thrive as a researcher. This will create tremendous respect for the profession and for that center as it will be seen on the cutting edge of chiropractic medicine. All this research can happen while increasing profits and further reaching broader bases of patients throughout your community.

Once all these steps are done in Phase 3, the last and final phase can be implemented.

Phase 4:

Phase four is simple, to continue growth in the community and expand this exact blueprint to similar cities within each state. Florida Hospital has different hospitals all over Florida, because it started with one hospital and grew to many different locations today. They can help people all over the state because their hospital had specific growth goals in mind. The same goes for these chiropractic centers. Begin by implementing this strategy in another city and then another, and then there could be chiropractic centers all over the world with high-level practitioners in each. All because one doctor decided to take these steps and course-correct the direction our profession is going.

This business model has been used before to great success within the medical profession. It is similar in how they went about expanding their outreach. The same must be done by chiropractic. Some may be fearful because the small cozy office is comfortable and growing into a large chiropractic center seems like too much work. That's fine by me, but there will be changes within the profession in the next 10 years, even if some chiropractors sit back and do nothing. The movement has already begun within the profession. You can choose to either sit back and do nothing while running yourself out of business or take this journey with me.

Daily Operations of these Centers:

Once a department is implemented, the practice would work off a very simple system. A proper patient intake system will be paramount to the success of this institution both financially and for patient care.

Typical patient flow

As a new patient enters a city's practice, they will be met by a front desk staff to get them properly logged into the system's computers. A resident of the General Chiropractic Division will meet the patient and escort them to a private room, where an extensive history and review of systems will be completed about their chief complaint. Vitals, general screening, a chiropractic exam and other special tests would be included to diagnose the patient. The resident's forms would then be reviewed by his head physician in his department and critiqued if needed. If the treatment could be completed by a general chiropractor, the patient would remain under the care of that resident and his head physician until resolved. If the diagnosis cannot be met or if the patient presents with a condition that would be better suited in another department, then the proper transportation of that patient to that department would be conducted to be reviewed by that department's director, practicing clinicians, and their residents. The patient's history and exam findings would be passed to that department electronically and care for that patient would be fulfilled by that department. This process will give the residents of the General Chiropractic Department quality diagnosing skills and will require an integrated and functional relationship between the departments.

Special patient flow

If a new patient presents to the clinic that is under 13, over 65, or has made an appointment with a specific department; they would be taken to the proper department by staff or greeted at the front by residents of that particular department. This would force residents to be patient-focused beginning from the initial encounter. Meeting the patients at the front would create a bond between doctor and patient that we would strive to promote throughout each chiropractic center. If a patient came to the practice with an obvious complaint to the residents of general chiropractic but had not made an appointment with the specific department, the resident would transport that patient to the proper department where an extensive and thorough history would be performed by a proper practicing physician. Relationships between departments will be active and encouraged to properly care for patients. Open lines of communication will be used to discuss and manage complicated cases, but also used for ease of referrals and co-managing of patients.

Returning Patients: a returning patient would be given to the doctor that had previously treated them. This could only change if the complaint has changed from a previous course of treatment. (Example: 1st CC-LBP, and 2 years later they have a stroke)

This center must be run by quality systems and conducted by professionals who are dedicated to seeing patients get better. Profits must be a side effect to our main goal, which is to get patients well under chiropractic care.

The center will be run under 8 Departments with a Director of each Department:

1. General Chiropractic
2. Neurology
3. Pediatric
4. Geriatric
5. Sports & Rehabilitation
6. Nutrition & Weight loss
7. Radiology
8. Research

Staff needed:

Doctors of Chiropractic

a. General Chiropractic Department
    i. Diversified
    ii. Gonstead
    iii. Upper Cervical

iv. Any other technique

b. Neurology

    i. Functional Neurology

    ii. Diagnostic Neurology

c. Pediatrics

    i. Pregnant mothers & Newborns

    ii. Kids up to age 13

d. Geriatrics

    i. Patients >65 years old

e. Sports & Rehabilitation

    i. Sports Performance

    ii. Personal Injury, Worker's Compensation

f. Nutrition & Weight Loss

g. Radiology

h. Research

Each of these departments would have a Director, who would oversee patient care and help with training of the residents in their departments. An attending physician would be implemented into each of these Departments when the need for expansion would arise.

Additional Staff:

1. Front Desk Associates
2. Insurance Professionals
3. Chiropractic Residents
4. Chiropractic Assistants
5. IT Professionals

The possibility of adding an Orthopedic Surgeon and a Family Practice Doctor would also be a priority since we would like to make our clinic a "one-stop shop" for all our patient's needs. With the high volume of patients that we would be seeing, undoubtedly, we would need an Orthopedic Surgeon on staff to help with complex cases that conservative care could not treat. However, any step that is taken to hire a new professional, must be approved by the Board first.

The first look at the beginnings of this facility should allow any chiropractor to visualize themselves being a much-needed member within this practice's model. The immensity of this idea is not possible for one person to undertake alone, which is why this is going to take a community of dedicated chiropractors that want to see their city healthier and with better access to holistic healthcare.

9

Possibilities after the change

Projections for each city

Each city is unique from any other city within the world and with it comes a set of challenges to overcome in setting up this unified chiropractic facility. The challenges could be not enough patients, no centralized location, low interest from other chiropractors, and the vastness of an undertaking this immense in each city. I am 100% committed to every state in the United States having these chiropractic centers strategically located throughout their cities. What is the perfect city for this model to work properly? Any city over 50,000 people that does not span more than 20 miles in any one direction, and has a minimum of 15 chiropractors ready to funnel their practice into a larger practice model. If a city meets these requirements than the probability for success goes astronomically higher. Let's do some projections, based on a sample city, to show the likelihood for success.

For this projection chapter, I will base all my calculations and reasoning on the average American city of 100,000 residents which is well-suited for this model. In a population of 100,000; there are approximately 12,000 chiropractic patients (12%). A city of 30 chiropractors are competing over these 12,000 patients, giving 400 patients per chiropractor to treat if dispersed equivalently. The average chiropractor with a patient base of 400, is paying for 2 other employees in his practice (front desk, chiropractic assistant). We are going to tackle how much money is spent on those employees per year and how much could be saved while under a unified chiropractic model. On average a front desk and chiropractic assistant are paid $12/hour. After payroll tax (135%) we will say that its approximately $16.20/hr. per employee. For a 40-hour work week, they are paid approximately $648/week and $2,805.84/month. With the two employees that you have, the total payroll comes to around $5,611.68/month. On average, each of chiropractor is paying that per month to keep his business functioning, since those employees are what keeps the business running day to day. With all 30 doctors on average paying that amount per month on payroll, the total would be $168,350.40/month for all these employees. If we chose to form a large group practice, the number of employees would decrease by a large amount. Only a select few of front desk employees would be needed and a talented group of chiropractic assistants would be needed to run the practice smoothly. For an example, let's say that we will utilize 4 front desk associates, 4 insurance professionals, and 15 chiropractic assistants. This would be total 23 employees, which would decrease the cost of payroll down to $64,534.32/month-a savings of $103,816.08/month. Over the course of a year's time that would save $1,245,792.96. That total alone would motivate me to want to integrate my practice with the other chiropractors in the city. That would save $28,619.57/per chiropractor.

When we discuss the possibility of sharing costs and expenses that number increases even more. If rent for a private practice were $1,500 there would be a total cost of $45,000/month going to rent all 30 buildings. Even if the building used to start the group practice is $30,000/month to rent, there would still be substantial increase in savings over the course of the year. The extra savings could be applied towards a variety of expenses, such as utilities, equipment, and office supplies. This would shave off unneeded spending throughout the month because it would be shared by the group of physicians.

One of the most important factors in grouping together would be the shared cost of marketing and advertising. For so long, each chiropractor has spent a few hundred dollars per month to market his practice to the community. With this shoestring budget, each one has tried the conventional advertising (TV, radio, newspaper) or the modern version of marketing (Facebook, Google, Instagram) to reach out to a target audience. With the restrictions to a budget, also comes restrictions in how many patients can see ads. With a group mindset to practice, we can add our marketing budgets together to get a tremendous response to each ad. This would allow mass advertising to the public, especially to people who have never even considered a chiropractor before. This would also give large amounts of exposure to our practice and increase the "hype" surrounding the start of this large center.

The projections for each city could be drastically different, especially in the large cities. The projections are staggering, though we would need to set up multiple groups across the vast area of those cities. Every city would have its challenges, but this is not a problem we can afford to put off till tomorrow, our profession needs it today.

Projections for Chiropractic Profession

This model is the future of the chiropractic profession, and each chiropractor needs to make the decision to be a part of it or not. We see all the signs pointing to group practice or integrated healthcare being beneficial to both patients and doctors. Doctors make more money with less stress, and patients get faster outcomes. Who wouldn't want that? Maybe some old-time chiropractors who like the way things were, but not this new generation. I know my generation wants change and are begging for things such as residencies and large centers in which to practice. Chiropractors have become complacent in their business strategies and that has carried over into the profession protecting our scope of practice. Just this year, Texas chiropractors almost lost their ability to function as a primary care provider and even losing the ability to treat the cornerstone of the chiropractic profession, the subluxation. Why is this happening to them? I believe it is because we have not banded together as a profession with regards to business strategies, and our communication within the profession is completely dysfunctional. If a basketball team doesn't communicate out on the court, they are going to lose. So many chiropractors have never met the other chiropractors within their own city. That is the reason there is dysfunction; because each chiropractor sees other chiropractors as competition and not as a teammate to help us reach our team goals. This is not a hard concept to grasp, but for so many chiropractors it has eluded them their entire careers. This new generation of chiropractors is hungry for change; I know, because I am one of them. I want to see our profession take the lead in healthcare and show the population how to truly be healthy. We have so much to offer, yet no platform in which to declare our benefits. That can all change with this model. We will then finally have the financial success within the profession to pursue meaningful research that furthers our claims as chiropractors, ease of communication within the profession to lobby for beneficial legislation within our government, and lastly build a team spirit within the profession that seeks to accomplish one goal-reach as many people with chiropractic care as possible.

10

The End of Private Practice

The medical profession is the most regulated profession in the United States. Nothing can move forward within healthcare because our government is choosing to pass laws that squelch any growth within medicine. MACRA is the newest threat that we face within chiropractic and all of medicine today.

The Medicare Access and CHIP Reauthorization Act (MACRA) is the newest form of legislation passed that is meant to incentivize outcome-based payments rather than our traditional fee-for-service model. Medicine grew accustomed to the Sustainable Growth Rate (SGR) and how physicians were paid for treatment of Medicare. SGR was not something that helped chiropractic by any means, but some practitioners could work within its requirements and make a decent living despite it. Now, with the advent of MACRA many chiropractors are fearful that it will be the end of the private practice.

MACRA started as a phenomenal idea within Washington D.C, and was conceptualized because of the over-treatment of patients on Medicare. This became a problem because under the fee-for-service model, the government felt that there was too much waste in spending on unneeded treatments and procedures for Medicare patients. They were 100% correct on this issue. Many doctors were gouging the system and were getting paid for unnecessary procedures, so the government had to step in and find an alternative. MACRA is that alternative they formulated, which seeks to pay for outcomes and results in medicine as opposed to treatments. This is a fantastic approach to medicine, but because the government is in control, there would be excessive amounts of paperwork and complying with regulations that doctors were not accustomed to before.

This compliance frightened chiropractors because we have already been under scrutiny, and many chiropractors believe this regulation to be the final straw that breaks the profession. Here's why so many doctors are saying that it could severely hurt the profession. We learned that 67% of chiropractors are in solo practice, and another 30% are in small group D.C practices, and with these new MACRA requirements those additional responsibilities would fall onto the solo doctor to comply with these standards. There are more outcome measures that each doctor must document and send to Medicare to make sure that they are reaching those standards or else they would get their reimbursements lowered by a percentage.

The four components to MACRA will focus 50% on the quality of care (similar to current PQRS), clinical practice improvement activities (CPIA). CPIA would allow chiropractors to choose from a list of practice goals that the practice much reach that year. The next component is cost, and if doctors can reduce the cost of care to patients, while still seeing similar outcomes of success. The final component replaces Meaningful Use (MU) and is called Advancing Care Information (ACI). Once doctors have reported all the data for each of these categories, it will get put into a formula to determine his/her Composite Performance Score (CPS). This score would then determine if the doctor would receive a penalty or a bonus for subsequent years with regards to Medicare reimbursement. These penalties or bonuses could range anywhere from 4-9% over the course of this new system, which could be a huge boost in revenue, or take even more money away from the minimal Medicare reimbursements already in place.

I have seen many consultants to chiropractors urging them to not participate in this program or to stop taking Medicare patients completely. They think that by avoiding the problem that it will just go away. This may be the dumbest advice they have ever given, because even if they ignore these new regulations they will still get a penalty in their reimbursements.

Other consultants are saying to use the provision built into this law, which allows for doctors who do not collect over $90,000 in Medicare reimbursements or do not see over 200 Medicare patients per year, to avoid having to comply with these requirements. I also find fault in this logic, because it breeds laziness from a business standpoint. To only shoot for $30,000 in reimbursements from Medicare, is like saying to a store to only sell a few pairs of shoes every year because we wouldn't want to work too hard this year. With that mindset, we are telling chiropractors to turn away patients because we do not want to deal with a proposal from the government. With the trend in insurance, whatever Medicare does first, the rest of the insurance companies will follow in like fashion. America is on a fast-track to socialized medicine, and Medicare was the first step to accomplishing that goal back in the 1900's. If we as chiropractors try to avoid being a part of this system, we will miss the opportunity to increase our outreach as a profession and will hurt the profession in the long run.

Complying with these standards can and will help chiropractic today. First, if we successfully comply and we generate amazing outcomes with our patients, we could be looking at a 4-9% increase in our reimbursements from Medicare. That may look insignificant, but it will compound over time, especially if we successfully put together these large group centers within chiropractic. That would take Medicare reimbursements in a large group practice from $250,000 to $260,000-$272,500, just for complying. Though not a large difference, over time these increase revenue streams would help the business grow in the future.

The second reason why I think chiropractic should participate in MACRA's requirements is that patients will be seeking a primary care doctor because their old one cannot see them anymore. Many medical doctors who have their own practice or work in a group of less than 15 are joining larger medical groups to make the transition with these requirements much easier. Some doctors are calling these measures "the death of primary care." This is pushing medical students into residencies and specialties far beyond primary care, which leaves a giant hole in the market for chiropractors to fill. All of these patients will need someone to perform their annual check-ups and physicals, and chiropractors are seated well to do just that. We cannot shy away from these patients because they are already feeling abandoned if their primary care doctors have left them. Taking the measures to fully comply would give us unparalleled access to patients, and we could expand our reach into homes that have never considered a chiropractor before.

These proposals could make the golden age of chiropractic if we are prepared for it, or it could absolutely destroy the profession if we choose to ignore it. The decision each chiropractor makes as a doctor will alter his/her outcome because there is no avoiding the crossroads we are facing today. A large group practice that I have proposed, led by The D.C Initiative, will have all the tools and necessary staff to successfully comply with the new MACRA guidelines. As a solo doctor, the choice to add another employee to help compliance, to personally do the work, or to avoid MACRA altogether. All these options severely diminish profits, increase stress, and reduce the ability to care for the patients we care about.

The D.C Initiative plans to set these supergroups together within chiropractic, because it will increase patient outcomes, streamline doctor's efficiency, and provide an administrative staff to handle all these new regulations with regards to insurance. These groups will increase profits, and will make one enjoy being a doctor because everything from a business standpoint would be handled. As a doctor, I cannot wait to see the positive effects these groups will have on my fellow colleagues and the patients we love so much.

11

Concerns & Conclusions

I understand this proposal has turned about 50% of you doctors and students completely off now that you are at the conclusion of this book. This dream of the future of chiropractic is a very polarizing idea, some of you will absolutely love it and some of you will absolutely hate it. I do not blame you for feeling that way; I'm glad you do! If everyone loved this idea, then there would be no push back on this plan, and it would probably have many flaws. Throughout writing this book, I asked countless colleagues about their take on this plan, many of them having constructive criticisms to it. I asked them for it, because I wanted perspectives from every part of chiropractic out there. I asked chiropractors from one side of the spectrum to the other for their creative insight, from subluxation-based philosophically driven practitioners to chiropractors who were open to having prescription rights in practice. It was in these conversations that I forged this idea to fit every chiropractor. It's far from perfect, but together we will work to perfect this idea so that every chiropractor finds his or her place in the future of chiropractic.

The next few pages I am going to address all the oppositional statements to this idea that I have heard over the course of writing this book. Each paragraph will address a different type of chiropractor or a different concern that each of you may have. I hope to iron out some areas for every single one of you, so that you can see the benefit that this model will have for our patients, and for ourselves.

First, allow me to address the practitioners who have their own private practice which is your "baby" and you never want to leave that practice you built. I completely understand that position. You have built that practice into something that is making a positive change within your community and you are very proud of it. You are the backbone of chiropractic today, if it wasn't for practitioners like you, patients would not have access to good quality chiropractic. As you work tirelessly to continue to reach out into your community and heal more patients, your time and energy has become switched from the beauty of chiropractic onto trying to grow your business. Though neither one of those is a bad thing, chiropractic has not progressed in breakthroughs in research and development. That is because all the chiropractors are focused on growing their business, not doing elaborate scientific experiments to prove/disprove theories and philosophies held dearly by chiropractic. Why have we not substantiated the subluxation to the world. We all know something is there and is affecting the nervous system, but we haven't proven in yet! This is because our best and brightest minds have been bogged down with running business that they may forgotten the beauty of chiropractic that enamored them in chiropractic school. This model gets our doctor's focus back onto patient care, which will drive copious amounts of data to be used for research and developing the future of chiropractic, all while the business is managed by a Board of Directors (who are still chiropractors--NOT BUSINESSMEN). Each of you chiropractors will become part owners in your city's chiropractic center and you will be able to choose the role that you want to play within this new model. If you want to pursue the business-side of the clinic, then that is your choice, but if you want to pursue breakthroughs in our profession than this will allow you to do just that.

The next problem that arose during conversations is that it will take too much work to form this massive endeavor in all these cities. Yes, that is correct. It will take a lot of work, but that is where my team at The D.C. Initiative steps in and makes this transition smooth and painless. There will be some things that you as a doctor must do in preparation for this transition, but the majority of the work will be handled by The D.C. Initiative, which will ensure that every willing chiropractor has a place in their city's chiropractic center. Our legal team will ensure a proper and ethical transition and that each chiropractor will be compensated based on the current value of their existing practice which is another incentive for those of you that already have a practice. As we evaluate your practice, the larger you are, the higher percentage of the center you will own, which means more authority and compensation from profits in the new clinic. This problem of being too much work has been completely thought out and completed by The D.C. Initiative's team of professionals.

Another big problem that I for see with a lot of practitioners is how would one chiropractor be able to work alongside other chiropractors that have completely different philosophies. That is a genuine concern, especially since there are so many different perspectives on how chiropractic benefits. Some may be purists of chiropractic and only treat the primary subluxation, and some of you may do the "Flying Seven" and every modality in the book. How could we all possibly get along and form a team and environment that promotes health and wellness. Here's how I see this problem within chiropractic today. Each of you that has their specific set of principles and ways that you treat patients are only seeing chiropractic from one perspective. Yes, you may get a vast majority of your patients well, but not every single patient that walks through your door gets better. What was missing with those patients that you couldn't get better? Perhaps, it was that you could only see that patient from one side of the problem or disease. Within this model, there will be a wide variety of practitioners who are treating patients within our center. This will create open communication channels between practitioners to know what other doctors have used to successfully treat with a different methodology. If a patient comes to see you with a problem that you haven't been very successful in treating, but you know that another doctor has been successful. The proper referral can be made so that patient can get better from the proper physician. It's always about the patient! Before, you would never refer a patient out to your competition, but now you are a team and teams must work together to be successful. Finally, I want to give you a final thought on this concept, if every player on your favorite sports team was the exact height and weight and had the exact same skill set as every other player, would that team be very successful? Now if it was Lebron James then maybe the argument could be made for that, but I'm not talking about outliers like him. As we are all very good at what we do, we fill in the holes that other teammates (doctors) have in their skill set, and they fill in holes that we have in our own skills. The synergy that could be formed when all chiropractors worked together towards a common goal would be phenomenal. We would be a force for good in every community, fighting against the traditional medical model of drugs and surgery that leave our patients helpless and without a cure for their condition. We are that chosen profession to do so, we just need to get along, this model would provide a way for that.

A logical question that arose was whether we make more or less money as chiropractors in this new model. I believe throughout the book I answered that question clearly. With sharing overhead expenses and increasing our reach to our communities, we will create revenues within the profession that we have not seen in the entire history of chiropractic. This would pay off in multiple ways. For those of you doctors who are on the front lines of these new centers, you would all be part owners in these centers. This will give you a portion of the profits every quarter to add onto your doctor's salary you are already getting. This will create incentive for all of you, like I have mentioned before. Then when you want to retire, you can sell your share in the company to an up-and-coming doctor. This would then create a passing-of-the-torch mentality to the next generation of chiropractors, which would give incentive for them to continue to make chiropractic profitable in the future. The profits from this clinic would also go towards forming Research and Development centers. These centers would then publish research that WILL validate everything we are doing in our clinics, which will drive more patients to come see our practitioners. The development of new technologies for our profession is also important, and these advancements could be funded in this business model, whereas they are unable to be funded presently. As the research and development is funded, the profession will be guided towards years of successful patient outcomes and successful advancements in medicine. Who said the only medical advancements have to come from medical doctors and Ph.D.'s? Let's get some D.C's the opportunity to make medical breakthroughs in treating conditions and diseases that have evaded us for too long. This model creates the potential for that to become a reality.

One of the last concerns I came across was eye-opening for me, because I had never thought about this before. One person said, "Mike, you are just in it for the money." As I walked away from that conversation, I had to really do some soul-searching to find what my true motivations were.

Yes, I wanted to make money to provide for my wife and family, but I passionately cared about the future of chiropractic. As I sought to find balance for my true motivations, I realized as I prayed and asked God to help me figure out this pressing question. I have come to peace with the fact that I do not care if I made a single cent from this entire business. I just want people to have unfettered access to the greatest form of healthcare this world has ever seen. I want every single person on this planet to get a taste of what true health is, and we as chiropractors are the agents of that change in the world. Throughout this whole process and as we go into the future, I want each of my fellow colleagues to know that I am aware of the billions of dollars in revenues that this model would create for chiropractic. I am not blind to that reality, but it is not my driving force. First and foremost, my motivation are to create a better future for chiropractic, a better future for our patients, and a better future for our world.

The last group I want to address are those students still in chiropractic school as all these changes are beginning in the profession. Many may think that there is no place for you in this model, but that couldn't be further from the truth. As the residency programs are officially launched within the profession, you will be the first applicants to go through these much-needed programs. We would validate our education with a formal residency program in each discipline that our centers must offer. This will give you many options in which to pursue a rich and fulfilling career. Many of you will become the leaders in the profession because some of us doctors that have been practicing for a while are already set on what path we want to follow. With this model, we would be able to provide both the resources and finances for you to make the groundbreaking medical discoveries this world needs. You will carry that baton into the future as we would continue to grow and develop chiropractic. Together, we would create a culture where patients could pursue true health in their lives and a world where the Doctor of Chiropractic becomes the leading healthcare expert. This world is only a few years away, will you be a part of it?

Contacting The D.C Initiative

Email: thedcinitiative@doctor.com

Phone: (850)776-3237

Twitter: @TheDCInitiative